Ketogenic Diet

Lose a pound a day instantly and become a fat burning machine

Kennedy Ross

KENNEDY ROSS

Additionally, the information in the following pages is intended only for informational purposes and should thus be thought of as universal. As befitting its nature, it is presented without assurance regarding its prolonged validity or interim quality. Trademarks that are mentioned are done without written consent and can in no way be considered an endorsement from the trademark holder.

Table of Contents

Introduction

Congratulations on purchasing this book and thank you for doing so.

The following chapters will discuss the basics of the Ketogenic Diet. This guide will explain how the diet works in detail, with tips and recipes to help you get started.

There are plenty of books on this subject on the market, thanks again for choosing this one! Every effort was made to ensure it is full of as much useful information as possible, please enjoy!

Chapter 1: How The Body Produces Energy

The body is an amazing machine. It turns every day foods we eat into energy that fuels the body. Each and every cell, from the brain and muscles, to skin and organs, need energy to perform everyday tasks that keep the body alive. Foods are all broken up into the three main macronutrients which are fat, protein and carbohydrates. Different types of foods have a combination of macronutrients, varying by their source. As each macronutrient is a physically different compound, the body must use different mechanisms to break them down into usable sources of energy.

The body's preferred source of energy is the carbohydrate, or also called sugars. They are quickly and efficiently broken down by the enzymes like lactase and amylase in the digestive system to be used as an immediate source of energy. Each type of sugar has a specific enzyme to break it down. This is evident in people with lactose intolerance. Lactose, a sugar from dairy products, is broken down by lactase. Those who are lactose intolerant do not have lactase, causing the lactose to pass through the digestive tract intact, causing a host of GI distress.

Not all sugars from carbohydrates are equal. Simple sugars, like refined white sugar and flour found in most baked products, is mostly broken down in the refining process, and therefore is absorbed and used very quickly. Complex sugars like unrefined grains with the husk intact, or starchy vegetables like sweet potatoes, require more work from the digestive system to break down, providing energy at a slower rate.

Plants contain sugars as well. Obvious sources like fruits are sweet and contain easily digested fibers, however, heavy fibers like cellulose from plants are considered sugars, but are not broken down at all. They simply pass through the gastrointestinal tract without providing any caloric benefit. How well a plant sugar is broken down depends on the thickness of the cell walls that make up the plant. The thicker the wall, the harder it will be for the body to digest. Plant fibers that do not provide any glucose at all are called insoluble fiber. While they provide no caloric benefit, they help keep the digestive tract moving. Water begins to flush into the intestines to flush out the indigestible material, quickening the transit time through the GI tract.

After ingestion, carbohydrates are broken down into single molecules of glucose, which are promptly processed by the liver, and enter the bloodstream. Hungry cells quickly take up most of the glucose provided by a meal. Each cell is capable of converting molecules of glucose into usable energy through a series of chemical reactions. While we will not discuss that entire process here, it takes several steps, and many other nutrients like vitamins and minerals to push that process along. The result is adenosine triphosphate (ATP), a direct energy source for the cell. Think of it like gas in a car.

The pancreas then releases insulin, a hormone that gathers excess glucose in the blood, and takes it back to the liver for storage. The liver can hold enough glucose for about two days worth of bodily function. Should you skip a meal and need a quick boost of glucose, glucagon, another hormone that regulates blood sugar, will prompt the liver to release some of its stored glucose into the blood stream.

Once the liver is full to its capacity, any excess glucose will be packaged and stored as fat. If excess amounts of glucose are consumed at every meal, the liver quickly runs out of room and molecules of fat begin to build up, something we familiarly call "gaining weight".

Proteins can be used for energy as well, but the body prefers to hold on to protein to maintain muscle mass. This is a mechanism that has been present in humans since the very beginning, and the reason behind it is very simple. The basic instinct in any human is the "fight or flight" response. It is ingrained in us to either run from our problems, or to stick around and defend ourselves. This was a primal instinct in our ancestors while they fought off predators, but still comes in handy as you try and catch the bus. Either way, you will need muscles to move your body. Your muscles would be weak and useless unless protein was there to keep them healthy and strong. Your body recognizes this, and puts priority into keeping your muscles ready at a moment's notice. When we think muscles, it is important to remember that the heart is a muscle, and the diaphragm that moves with your lungs are muscles, so this is not just for your arms and legs. This is basic physiological function.

Since proteins are so important, let's go through the sources. All animal products have protein. Meat from cows, pigs, chickens, eggs, and fish all have protein. A variety of plants, specifically the legume categories have protein too. All beans provide some protein, but as a plant, also have carbohydrates. Nuts and seeds also provide a good source of protein, along with fat. Almost all vegetables, including lettuce and tomato have small amounts of protein as well, but not enough to sustain the body as a primary protein source.

Proteins are not as easily digested as carbohydrates, and are therefore not the body's first choice of fuel source. It actually takes a bit more energy to digest a protein than a carbohydrate, so less of the calories in protein actually count since it takes energy to digest them. First, it takes more energy for the physical digestion, chewing, to happen in the mouth. A host of enzymes in saliva begin to work on breaking down the complex protein strings before it reaches the stomach, where most of the digestion occurs.

Proteins are broken down into amino acids, which are small enough to then enter the blood stream. Just as with glucose, amino acids circulating in the blood are quickly snatched up by cells that need them. While they serve a purpose in a number of ways in the body, muscle development and repair are their main function. Muscles are made of fibers called myofibrils, long strings of cells that run end to end of the muscle. Each muscle is made up of a large number of myofibrils. As we move our bodies, these muscle fibers stretch, contract, and break down. Once the muscle is resting, it can begin to repair any worn and torn fibers using amino acids from protein.

This process is the basis behind workout recovery. After a strenuous physical workout like lifting weights or running a marathon, the muscles become weak and tired, outside of their normal day to day wear. Many fitness experts recommend loading up on proteins to flush an abundance of amino acids into the muscles to speed recovery. Over time, the body adapts to the increased need for more muscle fibers to support the activity of the body. It builds more fibers and adds them to the muscle, so the weight of the activity is spread between more fibers. The result is a bigger, stronger muscle that can withstand longer workouts and more weight.

While the prospect of increasing lean body mass in muscles by consuming more protein, remember that anything in excess can actually be harmful. Just as with carbohydrates, any excess protein that the body cannot use in a timely manner will be stored as fat. So yes, protein can make you fat. On the other hand, too little protein will cause muscles to shrink. Proteins have many functional uses outside of muscles. Amino acids are essential for brain function and are part of the immune system response, both critical functions in the body. Remember that moderation is the key to keeping a balanced level of energy ready for the body.

Fats are also a great source of energy for the body. They, like protein, are complex molecules, and the body cannot readily absorb them like carbohydrates. While they are not the body's first choice in energy, they still account for almost half of the energy used by the body on a daily basis.

Fat is the most misunderstood macronutrient of all. With all of the negative press over the last few decades, fat has been reduced to the thing in our diet that makes us gain weight. This myth triggered a low-fat craze that lasted through the 1990's, prompting the development of low fat diet foods and several diet plans to banned fat. The general thinking was that fat is simply fat, and will be stored on our midsections and thighs. If it is eliminated from the diet, our waistlines would shrink.

The truth is much more complex. Dietary fat can come from a number of places. They are most abundant in animal products like beef, pork, chicken, eggs and fish. They are also found in plants like nuts, seeds, coconut, olive and avocado. There are several different types of fat that are used in the body in different ways. Saturated fats from animal products have been touted as killers in the past, as studies showed that they raised cholesterol and caused heart disease. While it is true that excessive amounts can lead to clogged arteries over time, saturated fat actually has a function in the body, and so getting at least a little in the diet is important. Saturated fats are required at a cellular level to facilitate communication between cells, and are an integral part in the body's natural fight or flight response.

Fats are broken down into smaller fatty acids by lipase, an enzyme produced in the pancreas. Fatty acids circulate through the blood attached to lipoproteins, LDL and HDL. You may recognize these as cells your doctor tests for to check your cholesterol. In fact, the quantities of each of these cells are a great indicator of what kinds of fat you are eating. For example, saturated fats that are synonymous with heart disease are carried around by LDL, or "bad cholesterol". The less saturated fat in the diet, the less LDL cholesterol will be circulating in the blood.

Good unsaturated fats from olive oil and avocado are carried around with HDL. It is important to have a low number LDL, indicating less saturated fat, and a high HDL, indicating a high amount of good fats. A high total cholesterol number will show that you have too much fat in your diet overall, and that the body is out of balance. Lab tests also test triglycerides (TG), which actually carry around carbohydrates meant for storage. A high TG number can be easily lowered by reducing carbohydrates in the diet.

Just as with any macronutrient in excess, large amounts of fat from the diet that cannot be used by cells immediately will be stored as fat. Once the fats have circulated, they get packaged to be stored as fat. Since the body's preferred source of fuel is carbohydrate, as long as the food you eat has both, the fat will be shunted toward storage for use later. The key is to eat at a calorie level that sustains your bodily functions, with little excess that will be stored for later.

On a larger scale, all fats are necessary in the digestive tract. Fat soluble vitamins like A, E, D and K can only be absorbed into the bloodstream if they are attached to a fat molecule. If you were to completely cut out fat, these vitamins would pass through the gastrointestinal system without being absorbed. Should this continue long term, the body would become deficient in these vitamins, causing issues with energy production, vision and blood clotting, all major functions of the body. They are also a main driver for hormone production in the body, which facilitates just about every major bodily function.

Fat is also a physical organ protector. Fat tends to accumulate around organs and cushions them, keeping them safe from trauma. It also acts as insulation to keep body temperatures up when hypothermia begins to kick in.

Chapter 2: What is Ketosis?

Chapter 1 tells us that pretty much everything we eat will be stored as fat unless it can be readily used by the body. This is an ideal scenario for the body, as its main goal is to keep you alive and prepare for later, not to look good in a bathing suit this summer. When food is scarce, the body is able to adapt and switch over to burning stored fat for energy, as there will be no carbohydrates coming in from the diet. The process of using stored energy is called ketosis.

During times where there are no carbohydrates available in the diet and carbohydrate stores have been depleted, fatty acids are released by the hormone glucagon from adipose (fat) tissue around the body, into the bloodstream. They are then sent to the liver where they can be converted immediately into usable energy, converted to ketones, which are an alternate source of fuel for the body. This process begins 2-3 days after a fast begins. At this point, the body has exhausted all of its glycogen stores in the liver, and must adapt to burn something else. Insulin production is dropped dramatically, allowing for the transition of fat for fuel.

Ketones can be utilized in all organs, including the brain, which was previously thought only able to run on glucose. It is a very efficient way to create energy without breaking down protein from muscles to use as energy. This saves valuable muscle strength to maintain the integrity of function while feeding the brain. Isn't the human body amazing!

The only factors that will stop ketogenic fat burning would be the reintroduction of carbohydrates, the body's preferred fuel, or once the fat stores are exhausted. The body will function this way as long as there is fat to burn in place of carbohydrates. Once all fat stores are utilized in a prolonged starvation situation, the body is forced to pull proteins from auxiliary muscles in the extremities to provide energy for crucial systems like the brain and other organs. The body would consider this a last resort to keep basic function going. Should muscle wasting occur to the point of decreased heart function, the person would be likely to die of starvation.

While most people can get through a bought of ketosis without any problem, sometimes a buildup of ketones can be harmful to the body. If functioning normally, the body can flush out excess amounts of ketones in the urine. A simple urine test can determine if the body is in ketosis by measuring the amount of ketones flushed out. However, too many ketones lingering in the body can cause ketoacidosis, a condition in which ketones remain in the blood and turn the pH acidic. This occurs when the body makes ketones at an unregulated rate, and the kidneys cannot process and rid the body of ketones fast enough. This is usually seen in Type 1 diabetics, in which there is a functional issue with the pancreas, and insulin, which shuts down ketone production, is not produced.

For most people, ketone production can be kept in check by small releases of insulin when levels start to become too high. It is recommended that people who have, or are at high risk for diabetes measure their urine ketone levels regularly to determine if they are present. It will be especially concerning if the person's diet includes enough carbohydrates to sustain the body, yet ketones are still being processed. This shows that insulin is not available to process the glucose, and dangerous medical conditions could be soon to follow.

Symptoms of ketoacidosis include stomach distress like nausea and vomiting, followed by decreases in brain function like confusion and blurred vision. If left untreated the patient could slip into a coma or even die.

While starvation is the worst case scenario, it is possible to maintain a state of ketosis without starving to death by only consuming a small amount of carbohydrates. While it varies by body size and genetics, keeping the diet under about 50 grams of carbohydrates per day will cause the body to burn fat out of necessity. Keep in mind that the body also relies on ketosis on a regular basis. Strenuous exercise, say running for an extended period or taking a class at the gym can deplete the liver's glycogen stores pretty quickly. That, plus the lack of oxygen to muscles due to increased needs puts the body in a fat burning mode during exercise. This period lasts about half hour after exercise while heart rate slows and breathing goes back to normal. During this time, fat is burned for energy.

Chapter 3: What is the Ketogenic Diet?

The Ketogenic Diet is an eating plan that is meant to maximize the body's fat burning potential by keeping the metabolism in ketosis. The body can be programmed to burn only fat, based on the things it is fed. While ketosis is meant to be a survival mechanism for the body, we can use this to our advantage. By only burning fat, excess body fat will decline, leading to overall weight loss.

The idea is simple. Change the ratio of macronutrients fed to the body to be mostly fat and protein, with minimal carbohydrates. In this diet, carbs and sugar are eaten more like condiments, in small amounts. About 70% of calories should be from fat, about 25% from protein and about 5% from carbohydrates. The exact number of grams of carbohydrates will vary by the person, and the calorie content of the diet overall.

While you should consult a health care professional to determine what calorie level and carbohydrate level is right for you, most of the time, carbohydrate levels fall between 30 and 100 grams per day. In general, people who exercise regularly can stand to tolerate more carbohydrates, as they will burn through them quickly enough to remain in ketosis.

The Ketogenic Diet was first developed back in 1924, at the Mayo Clinic by Dr. Russell Wilder. The eating plan was created to help epileptic patients manage and eliminate their seizures. It is not fully understood why seizures diminish with the metabolic shift, but decades of research shows that there is a direct correlation.

The diet lost steam in the 1940s as several medications were developed to treat seizures. Taking medications was much easier than following a strict diet that limited food choices. The Keto Plan re-emerged in the 1970's when Dr. Irwin Stillman published *The Doctor's Quick Weight Loss Diet.*

Dr. Stillman worked with weight loss patients in Brooklyn, New York. He found that weight loss occurred quickest when his patients followed a low carb, high lean protein diet. He supported a diet based on lean proteins like skinless chicken, seafood, eggs and low fat cottage cheese. The strict regimen eliminates all sugars, fruits, vegetables and most fats. Alcohol was off limits.

One major downfall, besides the lack of imagination in food choices, is the nutrition content is heavily imbalanced. Common knowledge tells us that fiber, vitamins and minerals only found in fruits and vegetables is strictly off the diet. Staying on the plan for a prolonged length of time will lead to nutritional imbalances and deficiencies. Dr. Stillman recommended supplements to meet nutritional needs while on the diet for extended periods of time.

He claims, however, that his patients trended to lose 10-15 pounds in the first week alone, then about 5 pounds per week thereafter. He did not recommend staying on this diet for weight maintenance once the goal weight was met. Transitioning back to a well balanced, calorie controlled diet was most beneficial for maintaining weight and nutrient status.

More modern versions of the Keto diet utilize very low carb vegetables as part of the plan to make sure vitamins, minerals and fiber are consumed. This modification makes it more reasonable to stay on the diet for a longer period of time without the need for supplementation. Low carb vegetables can be eaten in proper portions to stay within carb limits for the day.

More extreme versions of the Keto Diet also exist. Two versions, the Targeted Ketogenic Diet (TKD) and the Cyclic Ketogenic Diet (CKD) are meant for people who are very physically active and can fully commit themselves to the diet. This is usually reserved for professional athletes and body builders, but anyone with a strong commitment to diet change can learn to utilize these versions.

The Targeted Ketogenic Diet pairs carbohydrates with exercise. In this plan, eating around 25grams of carbohydrates just before exercise gives the body the immediate energy it needs to complete the physical task of exercise, yet is consumed by the body so quickly that the over ketosis system is not affected. Once the workout is complete, the carbs are gone, and the body goes back into ketosis. It is recommended to refuel with a high protein low fat and low carb meal after exercise for recovery.

While the theory behind this method is good, more recent research suggests that the body actually performs better during exercise under a ketogenic metabolism, and consuming carbs right before a work out can make the body sluggish.

Remember that about 25 grams of carbs equals about two slices of bread, or 2 cups of fruit. Strenuous exercise after a heavy meal like this may hinder performance.

The Cyclic Ketogenic Diet focuses on carb loading on certain days of the week, rather than just before exercise. Most plans recognize that carb loading for 2 of 7 days is beneficial to maintain physical performance while burning fat for 5 days a week on a keto plan. Carb loading usually means eating about 500 grams of carbohydrates on a carb loading day. To put this in perspective, this would equal about 15 cups of pasta or 20-30 cups of fruit in one day. While this may seem like a carb-lover's dream, this amount of carbohydrate in such a short time will likely lead to stomach upset, constipation and nausea. To keep up this plan on a regular weekly basis is unrealistic, to say the least.

The general consensus is that staying on a standard Ketogenic Diet brings the most success as compared to the strictest Keto plans. Changing the meal plan to include about the same ratio of carbohydrates, protein and fat on a daily basis keeps ketosis in place without causing any unnecessary stress on the body. Meals can easily be planned around the same framework, and does not require eating excessive amounts of food on selected days of the week. When followed correctly, weight loss occurs with little effort, and with little hunger throughout the day. More detailed directions for getting started will be available in Chapter 7.

Is this diet right for you? Lots of people have a very hard time sticking to any diet, and the Keto plan really will be no different unless you are truly ready to change some dietary habits. No diet will work unless you are able to commit. With the Keto diet, a high level of commitment is required on a daily basis in order to maintain the constant metabolic process of ketosis. The body would willingly switch back over to burning carbohydrates as soon as it gets the chance, so having one or two highly carb-based meals per week will disrupt the fat burning process, hindering your results. Carbohydrates trigger the release of insulin, and as long as it is present in the blood, the body will stay out of ketosis, and no fat will be burned.

If you plan to begin this diet, make sure you are prepared to stick to it for the best results. Just know that the small sacrifices you make will lead to lasting results and better health. This means creating a plan of action for your meals and getting organized. Put in the prep work now for easy, continued success later.

What is NOT allowed on a Ketogenic Diet?
The nice thing about the Ketogenic Diet is that, by default, it eliminates most problem foods we see in today's food market. Carbohydrates run rampant in most packaged, processed foods. Automatically eliminated are cookies, crackers, breads and sweets. All other legitimate diets will probably do the same.

The majority of dairy products will also be eliminated, due to their sugar content. A cup of whole milk has about 15 grams of carbohydrates, about a third of the carbohydrate limit for the day. While it is possible to work it in, it will unlikely be a staple in your diet. Fat free milks actually contain higher sugar contents in order to make up for the missing fat. Just forget all about chocolate milk!

For the most part, fruits will also be eliminated on this diet. Fruits with high water content, like watermelon and strawberries, can be eaten in moderation, but should not be a staple in your diet. These varieties average about 15g of carbohydrate per cup, so adding them sparingly here and there could work. Sweeter fruits like ripe bananas contain about 30 grams of carbs each, and will likely not work in the plan. It's safer to eliminate fruits altogether, as eating a concentrated amount of sugar at once during the day may shift your metabolism out of ketosis.

What CAN I eat on a Ketogenic Diet?
The list of excluded foods is actually pretty small. The door is open on all proteins, all fats and most vegetables. Let's go through them for a little more clarity.

For this diet, focus on getting your protein from meat sources like chicken, fish, beef, pork and eggs. These sources of protein contain only protein and fat. Do not rely on meatless sources of protein like beans and tofu for protein, as any plant-based protein will also contain carbohydrates. It will be easy to go over your carbohydrate limit for the day if your proteins are sourced from plants. For example, a half cup serving of black beans packs 21 grams of protein, but also 60 grams of carbohydrate! The beans may be filling, but you can kiss ketosis goodbye.

Make all of your proteins lean. Fatty cuts of meat like bacon are fine in moderation, just as in any diet. High fat meats are rich in cholesterol raising saturated fat, which can increase your risk for heart disease. Choose lean cuts of meat like chicken and fish, and leave the fats to added unsaturated oils like olive or avocado.

This diet focuses on getting energy from fat, therefore, fat in the diet is encouraged, however, the type of fat matters. As we discussed earlier, healthy polyunsaturated fats should be eaten the majority of the time. Good sources of healthy fats include olive oil, coconut oil and avocado. Just remember that you will also need to stay within a modest calorie limit to prevent excess calories being converted for fat storage. Oils and fats pack a lot of calories into a small amount, so be sure to watch your portions.

Let's get down to carbohydrates. All traditional carbs like rice, potatoes and pasta are off limits on a Ketogenic Diet. What we need to be careful of is vegetables that contain carbohydrates in small numbers, yet add up quickly. Most leafy green vegetables are safe to eat in abundance. About a cup of romaine lettuce has only about 1 gram of carbohydrate. Go ahead and load up your salad. Be a little more careful with tomatoes and peppers, which have higher carb content, about 5 grams per cup. Higher still is broccoli, carrot or onions which come in at about 12 grams per cup. While these vegetables are healthy to include in your diet every day, just watch your total carbs. Your best bet will be to pair some very low carb with some moderate carb vegetables to maintain your levels.

How do you know you are in ketosis?

There are subtle signs to know you may have reached ketosis. First off, give your body a few days on the new diet to burn off stored glucose and to switch the metabolism to ketosis. Do not measure your success of entering ketosis until this time has lapsed. After a few days, you may notice a sweet aroma to your breath, almost a fruity fragrance. This is a common side effect of ketosis, as ketones themselves are sweet. While the condition isn't harmful, it may alter how you taste things, a small annoyance. This usually disappears after a week or two on the diet.

Another common symptom is the frequent need to urinate. While this can also correlate to an increase in fluid, the breakdown of glycogen in the liver causes more need for the kidney to produce urine, causing it to be excreted more often. As glycogen stores deplete, this symptom is likely to subside.

Some people get a lightheaded or dizzy symptom, especially when beginning a new diet. This correlates directly to the increase in urination. As the kidney works to get rid of excess byproducts of glycogen breakdown, it also eliminates electrolytes and minerals like potassium, sodium and magnesium. Low levels of any of these can cause you to feel fatigued, almost like you just exercised and lost them through sweat. These deficits may make you feel dizzy or give you headaches and leg cramps. As glycogen stores deplete and ketosis is reached, these symptoms usually decline.

For the most part, the side effects reported with following the Ketosis Diet are limited to the transition stage of the diet as the body makes preparations to change the metabolism to its fat burning mode. To reiterate again, if you have underlying health conditions, specifically diabetes, consult a health care professional before beginning a Ketogenic Diet, and report even small side effects to your doctor. Diabetics could enter ketoacidosis, a potentially deadly metabolic condition, and should be monitored very closely should they want to try this diet.

The certain way to know if you are in ketosis at any given time is to measure the ketone levels in your urine. Ketone test strips are available at most major pharmacies without a prescription. The test can be done in one of two ways. Either pass the test strip under a steady stream of urine, or collect a small sample and dip the strip in. Either way, wait about 15 seconds for the reaction to occur. If you are not in ketosis, the test strip will remain a beige color. If the strip changes color, use the guide on the test strip box to determine what level of ketosis you are in.

Most strips show a darker blue or purple color to indicate the highest number of ketones in the blood. It isn't always necessary to get the highest number, as some people burn fat more efficiently at more moderate ketone levels. Since this is highly variable depending on the person, test your ketones regularly and compare to how you feel and at what rate you are burning fat to determine the optimal level for you.

Log your daily numbers and food choices in a notebook, especially during the beginning phase of your diet. After awhile, you will begin to recognize trends in your ketone numbers based on the meals you have eaten, and you will know what foods will keep you at a steady ketone level. Until you get it write it down.

A downfall to this ketone test is your hydration level. You may have noticed that when you are thirsty, or have not had much to drink during the day, that your urine is a dark yellow color. The color indicates concentrated levels of urea and waste exiting the body. On the other hand, when you are well hydrated, urine is much lighter, almost clear, indicating that most of the waste being eliminated is excess water. If you are very hydrated, your ketones will be much more diluted in the urine, which could make your test seem like you are not in ketosis. The opposite is also true if you are dehydrated and your ketone levels are unexplainably high.

Pay attention to your hydration status by checking urine color and mentally correct for discrepancies. To avoid this skewing your results often, try to drink a consistent amount of water every day, and do the ketosis testing a couple times a day, once in the morning when you are least hydrated, and once at night when you will likely be more hydrated.

Why not cut out ALL carbs?

First off, it really is not practical to cut out all carbohydrates. Remember that Dr. Stillman's Diet did cut out all carbohydrates, including vegetables. Not only was the adherence rate to the diet low, the plan itself was nutritionally off balance. Vegetables do have small amounts of carbohydrates, which need to be monitored, but they also contain fiber, vitamins and minerals that are not found in protein and fat sources on this diet. Adherence to this strict diet long term would lead to nutritional deficiencies and the need for supplementation. The lack of fiber would slow the digestive tract motility leading to constipation, bloating and discomfort. Low fiber diets, unless therapeutically warranted, carry a higher risk of intestinal cancer due to the chronic decreased motility. For this reason, we keep low carb vegetables in the diet.

Another long-standing reason why some carbs are still included in the Ketosis Diet is the notion that red blood cells and vital organs like the brain and liver require glucose to function properly. One side effect of ketosis, usually at the beginning, is mental fatigue. Early studies showed that the brain functioned better and faster when glucose was metabolized for energy, and slower under ketosis.

Newer research is showing that the theory isn't correct, reason being that the body has developed ketosis as a means of survival, and using a fuel source that would not work in the brain is basically useless. The brain is the starting point for all of the body's function, and without it, ketosis would not be necessary to power the rest of the body. While study results are inconclusive and require further testing for a definitive answer on that, we will still include vegetable carbs in the Keto Diet, for all of the other reasons listed above.

Chapter 4: Benefits of the Ketogenic Diet

Now that we have covered the science behind metabolizing fat through ketosis, we can discuss the health benefits of doing so. While the mechanism of ketosis is meant as a means of survival for the body, the benefits to our health really stand out.

As this e-book focuses on, the Ketogenic Diet is great for weight loss, especially weight from excess body fat and stored water weight. Especially at the beginning of ketosis, the body rids itself of excess water molecules that typically attach themselves to sugars and salt that are quickly excreted by the kidneys. As glycogen stores are diminished, excess sodium is flushed out with the byproduct of glycogen metabolism, and water weight diminishes. The majority of weight loss in the early stages of ketosis are from excess liquid that makes you feel bloated and heavy. Your blood sodium levels will also decrease, eliminating water in the blood vessels, lowering blood pressure as well.

Studies show that dieters following a low carb plan lose more weight versus those following a low fat diet at the same calorie levels. On top of that, low carb plan followers report feeling less hungry than low fat dieters, making it much easier to adhere to the diet over time. Fat and protein are not as quickly broken down by the body, and remain in the digestive tract for longer periods of time. This leaves you feeling fuller, longer than a high carb, low fat diet.

Studies also show that most of the fat lost on a low carb diet is from the abdominal region, which has a higher amount of visceral fat. Visceral fat is that which surrounds organs, and in excess, causes pressure and strain on them, creating health problems. As visceral fat is lost, the waist line decreases and the risk for chronic diseases diminish.

Ketosis also spares protein from muscles being burned from fuel. Since most people who diet would prefer to lose fat and gain muscle, this is the perfect diet. The body will adapt to burning fat only, and protein from the diet will be used to build and repair muscles, rather than for energy.

One of the first benefits realized with the Ketogenic Diet is with epilepsy, a condition whose sufferers deal with uncontrolled seizures. Patients with epilepsy are limited by their condition, often needing help doing everyday tasks like driving, for fear of having an epileptic episode while driving.

Studies have yet to pinpoint exactly why ketosis reduces and even eliminates symptoms in some patients, but they conclusively see correlations with decreased seizures in patients on a Ketogenic Diet. Studies reported by the Epilepsy Foundation show that half of pediatric patients on the diet reduce the occurrence of seizures by fifty percent, some even become seizure free. While it is not recommended to stop or reduce prescribed epilepsy medications due to reduced seizures, the Ketogenic Diet is a great compliment to current medication regimens.

Because the Ketogenic Diet has worked wonders on epileptic patients, research is being conducted to find out if following the diet will benefit patients with diseases like Alzheimer's disease and Parkinson's disease, which largely affect the brain.

The Ketogenic Diet does wonders for diabetes and elevated blood sugar levels as well. While it is extremely important to monitor symptoms of ketoacidosis, the elimination of most carbohydrates reduces the need for insulin, the main functional issue seen in diabetes. Those who have elevated blood sugar levels or are on the verge of developing diabetes will most definitely benefit from decreasing sugars and carbs in the diet. Type 2 diabetes develops when the diet is out of check. High intake of carbohydrates exhausts the mechanisms that produce insulin, the hormone responsible for processing and storing excess glucose.

As sugars flood the system, the body becomes insulin resistant, leaving excess glucose circulating in the blood. The crystalline structure of sugar causes damage to blood vessels, destroys nerve endings and leads to several other related diseases, including heart disease. Diabetics commonly suffer from decreased feeling in their extremities due to decreased blood flow, and damage to blood vessels in the eyes, causing blindness if left unchecked.

The Ketogenic Diet eliminates excess carbs in the diet, lowering blood glucose levels, and decreasing the need for insulin. Patients who follow a low carb diet will see their blood glucose numbers drop, and will stop the progression of diabetic symptoms.

Despite what you may think, following a low-carb diet plan will decrease your triglyceride numbers. All other cholesterol markers are measures of fat quantity and quality in the diet; however, triglycerides are directly affected by the amount of carbohydrates in the diet. Lowering the carbs will reduce those numbers your doctor has been hounding you about.

Speaking of cholesterol numbers, following this diet correctly should also change the ratio of LDL (bad cholesterol) to HDL (good cholesterol). Eating lean meats that are low in saturated fats and concentrating on better unsaturated fats like olive oil will lower your bad LDL cholesterol and increase your good HDL cholesterol. Your risk for heart disease will decrease and your doctor may reconsider putting you on cholesterol lowering medications.

The Ketogenic Diet is also being studied with cancer patients. There is lots of new research suggesting that cancerous cells and tumors like to feed off of glucose exclusively, just like your body. While your body has mechanisms to adapt to ketosis, cancer cells do not, Cutting off the power source for a cancerous tumor can cause it to weaken, shrink, and become more susceptible to treatment. This is an interesting line of thinking, and may be used in coordination with chemotherapy treatments and surgery to increase the patient's chance of survival.

Chapter 5: The Keto Diet compared to other popular diets

Why choose the Ketogenic Diet over other popular diets? The short answer is no other diet changes the body's metabolism to utilize ketosis exclusively. Some diets come close, lowering carbohydrate levels drastically, but coming just short of ketosis. Let's take a look at some of today's most popular diets.

The Atkins diet is the most recognizable low carb diet out there right now. The Atkins diet was developed by cardiologist Robert C. Atkins in the early 1970s. It was meant to help his patients with heart conditions lose weight and decrease their risk of complications of heart disease. The main focus is cutting out carbohydrates from grains like bread, pasta, oatmeal and rice, the traditional carbohydrates.

Unlike the Ketogenic Diet, there are several phases to the Atkins diet, making it much more complicated to follow. Phase 1 of Atkins is similar to the Keto Diet, restricting carbohydrates to 20 grams of net carbs per day. Followers are urged to make their plate mostly vegetables (within the carb limit), lean protein and healthy oils. This phase lasts about two weeks

Phase 2 of Atkins, followers stay at 12-15 grams of carbs, then slowly add back carbs via bigger portions of vegetables, and adding some low sugar fruits. Phase 2 should result in about a

10 pound weight loss, and it is recommended to stay in Phase 2 until this goal has been reached.

In Phase 3, the follower adds back about 10 grams of carbs back to the diet per week. At this point, weight loss must be carefully monitored against the carb level. If weight loss stops, too many carbs have been added back. Once the goal weight is reached, it is important to maintain a low level of carbs to avoid weight from creeping back up.

Unlike the Ketogenic Diet, Atkins has developed a line of approved Atkins foods including drinks, protein bars and frozen meals to help their followers keep on track. The Keto Diet, in contrast, uses real foods that are found everywhere as the basis for the plan. While it is possible to do the same thing Atkins, lots of their followers get accustomed to simply picking Atkins approved foods, and when they get bored, have a hard time figuring out how to transition

The Blood Sugar Diet, developed by Michael Mosley is a low carb spin on the traditional Mediterranean Diet. The Mediterranean Diet focuses on the diet of a group of people in Italy and other countries surrounding the Mediterranean Sea. These people traditionally had much lower incidence of disease, prompting the development of a diet that mimics their eating habits. The traditional diet does utilize carbohydrates from fruits and whole grains, and does not really set a carbohydrate level to stay under. Mosley's plan takes a carb limit into account and recommends limiting the total number of calories to 800 per day, as part of an initial fast. This cuts carbs by necessity. The fast should last about 8 weeks, at which time a 2 day per week fast will be implemented. The driving force behind Mosley's plan is to drastically reduce blood sugar and stave off diabetes. Weight loss does occur as a result.

Mosley's low carb plan is different from the Keto Diet because it allows traditionally Keto eliminated carbs like low sugar fruits, legumes and dairy. This diet may induce ketosis in some people, depending on their body's threshold for carbohydrates, but may not in others. Followers will likely lose weight due the calorie restriction, but 800 calories is a very hard level to maintain. Most people need a minimum of 1500 calories a day just to sustain basic body functions, let alone participate in exercise. At low calorie levels, the brain constantly focuses on food, and it may be much more difficult to manage this diet.

The Keto Diet does not recommend a strict calorie restriction, but limiting calories only to your daily needs, not in excess. An active adult will average 1800 to 2500 calories depending on age, weight, gender and activity level. This is enough to enter ketosis, yet keep the body and brain full and satisfied.

The Paleo Diet is similar to the Ketogenic Diet in a number of ways. The Paleo Diet, developed by Dr. Loren Cordain, based on studies spearheaded by Dr. Alessio Fassano focuses on the diet of our ancestors, before modern agriculture and domestication of livestock. In short, Cordain explains that agriculture and the introduction of previously uneaten foods has developed very quickly, and that our bodies have not evolved to tolerate them as readily. As a result, certain foods cause harm to the digestive tract, triggering the immune system. Inflammation throughout the body occurs, leading to autoimmune diseases and weight gain, especially if complimented with small excesses in calories.

The idea is to cut out inflammatory foods like gluten and dairy, which happen to be eliminated on the Keto Diet as well. While the reasoning behind removing these foods is different between diet plans, the result is the same decrease in blood sugar, and less storage of fat. The Paleo Diet does not specifically limit carbohydrates, but does model meals around lean proteins and non-starchy vegetables. Starchy vegetables like sweet potato and winter squashes, as well as fruits are allowed. It eliminates starchy legumes for inflammatory reasons. Followers may reach ketosis, but are unlikely to maintain it constantly on the Paleo Diet unless carbs are specifically limited.

Chapter 6: Exercise and the Ketogenic Diet

Every good diet comes with an effective exercise plan. Several sources report that exercising isn't necessary on a Ketogenic Diet, and this is true, in a way. The benefits of the diet include feeling less hungry throughout the day, decreasing the daily calorie amount, which will lead to weight loss. With a Keto Diet, most weight lost is fat, and total weight loss does happen pretty quickly.

The same is true for other calorie restricting diets, yet fat burning does not happen as readily without cardio exercise, and it takes about fifteen minutes of cardio before the body enters a fat burning mode. Ketosis has the body burning fat all the time, so there is no delay with exercise, the body will simply increase the rate of fat burning to provide for increased energy needs.

The bottom line is, if calories are in a deficit for extended periods of time, weight loss will occur, it will just happen at a slower rate. This is good news for people who do not have the physical capability to exercise at this point due to extreme obesity or other medical conditions, but will be able to incorporate activity as their weight decreases. However, results can be improved by incorporating exercise.

In order to lose about a pound per day on the Ketogenic Diet, regular exercise is recommended, if your doctor deems you fit enough for activity. To begin, take possible side effects of transitioning to ketosis in mind. If starting the diet makes you lethargic or light headed, consider refraining from exercise until those symptoms subside. This would be especially true if you are not used to exercising, as doing something strenuous may make those symptoms worse. Once you feel comfortable continuing your exercise program or stepping into a new one, go ahead and get started.

There are many other health benefits to regular exercise, as your doctor has likely told you. Increasing cardio exercise is crucial to cardiovascular health. When you work your heart, it becomes stronger and more efficient, just as with any muscle. Blood is able to circulate more efficiently, and your stamina increases. Benefits of better cardiovascular health can be seen every day. You will not wear out as quickly, will have more energy, and will be able to climb stairs and walk around with ease. As you increase the well being of your heart, you reduce the risk of heart disease, which could prolong your life.

Cardio workouts and weight lifting both strengthen muscles throughout the whole body. Consistent exercise regimens result in bigger, stronger muscles with much more capability to work. Whether you work in a warehouse and lift all the time or work a desk job, increased muscle strength will be useful everywhere.

Even better, increased muscle mass increases the number of calories you burn throughout the day. It actually takes more energy to maintain, grow and repair muscle mass than it does to maintain fat stores. By increasing muscle mass with exercise, you are increasing your strength and increasing your daily calorie burn, even at rest. Just don't get carried away. Yes, your muscle will burn more calories, but averages only another fifteen calories per pound of muscle mass gained. This isn't a license to eat more, especially if you are still trying to reach your weight loss goal. It is however, a nice perk.

Regular exercise also decreases the risk of diabetes and reduces insulin resistance. Combined with a Ketogenic Diet, this is a great way to avoid diabetes. Several studies over time have shown that regular exercise, especially aerobic, like jogging or running lower blood sugar levels, and decrease insulin resistance. This means that the body can normally respond to glucose in the blood by releasing an appropriate amount of the hormone insulin, which filters excess glucose to the liver to be stored for energy. This benefit of exercise, plus the low carb aspect of the diet itself is a double whammy against the development of diabetes.

Exercising on a regular basis also improves mood, energy and decreases the risk of brain related diseases like dementia. It is well known that exercise boosts the mood by releasing endorphins, or good feeling chemicals in the brain. This effect lasts for a good part of the day, increasing mood overall. Exercise also helps regulate neurotransmitters related to sleep, resulting in better, more restful sleep. Several studies have shown that people who exercise regularly have a decreased risk of age related mental disease, like Alzheimer's. It seems that exercise keeps the brain fresh, slowing the aging process within the brain

As you begin to develop an exercise plan for yourself, don't just think about the weight loss and improvements to your physique. Studies show that people who begin exercise for vanity tend to lose interest in their plan quickly. Those who focus on more health related goals tend to stick with it longer. The theory is that the prospect of better health will extend life, and improve quality of life.

It is also important to find activities that you enjoy doing. Some people really enjoy going to the gym, running on the treadmill and lifting weights on a regular basis. Others wouldn't be caught dead there, and would prefer hiking, running or biking outside. This is really a matter of preference, but studies show that people will maintain regular exercise if they actually like what they are doing. If you are just contemplating an exercise plan, do some research.

Try different activities and classes, and experience workouts at different gyms before committing to a membership. Consider factors like proximity to your home and convenient locations when trying to choose a gym, but also the atmosphere. If you do not feel comfortable at a particular gym, you will be less likely to continue going there. Don't feel like you need to continue one type of activity exclusively. Lots of people label themselves as runners or bikers, and that's because they truly enjoy those things. If you get bored with a routine or don't think it is working for you any more, change your routine and try something else.

Where you start with an activity plan depends on your current fitness level. Consult with your doctor to make sure you are fit enough for the activity you plan to do, and for advice for where to start. It's okay to ease into a new routine. Even if you are doing a little more than you were before, you are ahead of the game. Keep in mind that sticking to your diet will have the biggest impact on your weight and health. Focus on getting that right, then add exercise once you feel comfortable with the plan.

Chapter 7: How To Get Started

By now, you may be feeling overwhelmed, wondering how you should get started. After all, attention to detail is important to entering and maintaining ketosis. Here are a few guidelines to get you started.

Rule # 1: Stick to 30-100 grams of net carbohydrates per day. Note that there is a distinct difference between net carbs and total carbs. Net carbs are simply the amount of total carbs minus the amount of fiber. While grams of fiber are technically carbohydrates, remember that they pass through the gastrointestinal system nearly intact. None of the carbs actually get digested and used, so they cannot count toward carbohydrates.

Knowing the difference between total carbs and net carbs will be a helpful tool, and opens up the door for larger amounts of vegetables, which will keep you fuller, longer. Simply check the nutrition facts label on your foods and subtract the grams of fiber from the total carbs to figure out the net carb content. Unfortunately, not all vegetables have labels, so you may need to rely on the internet for that information. Websites like SELF Nutrition Data allow you to enter just about any type of food to get a nutrition label.

Rule # 2: Determine an appropriate calorie level for balance.

Finding a good balance of calories is important for any diet plan. Too little calories will leave you feeling hungry, tired and weak. If your calorie is level is too low for too long, your body may resort to pulling protein from muscles for energy, decreasing muscle mass, which is probably not the look you're going for. Too many calories, even from fat, will be stored as fat for energy use later. While your body may be losing fat in ketosis, excess calories from the diet will quickly replace those burned, and weight loss will be slowed, if it even budges at all.

Rule # 3: Test for ketones and compare to your meal choices.

The only certain way to find out if you have reached ketosis is to test your urine for ketones. Investing in test strips and testing a couple of times daily, especially in the beginning, will help you determine if your body is producing ketones. Keep a written log of your ketone levels alongside your meal choices for the day. You will start to see correlations to higher carb meals and lower ketone levels.

You will quickly determine what your ideal carbohydrate levels are for your body, which will help you pinpoint an ideal fat burning diet for you. Because ketosis varies by person, by specific diet and activity level, doing a little experimentation is a good way to get it right without the guesswork.

Rule # 4: Monitor any side effects

This rule is important for diabetics or for those who may be susceptible to ketoacidosis, a serious and potentially fatal condition. Aside from ketoacidosis, people react a little differently to a changing meal pattern. Some may be more sensitive, having bouts of dizziness and fatigue that could be bothering and possibly harmful. Incidences of faintness, quickening heart rate and shortness of breath have been reported, so it may be a good idea to limit strenuous exercise, at least for few days to determine what effect transitioning to ketosis may have on you. Should you have any concern for your health, go back to your original diet plan immediately, and consult your doctor.

Chapter 8: Recipes

Now that you know the ins and outs of the Keto Diet, use the following recipes to get started. This delicious collection follows the recommended carbohydrate limit for each meal, which will be enough to get most people into ketosis quickly. Remember that the carbohydrate levels at which ketosis begins differs by person. These recipes will work for almost everyone, but check your ketone status regularly to make sure your diet is effective.

Breakfast Ideas

Avocado Bacon and Eggs
Serves 1
Ingredients
1 slice of turkey bacon
1 small avocado
2 eggs
1 tbsp cheddar cheese
½ tsp salt

Instructions
Preheat oven to 425°F.

Cut the ripe avocado in half, remove the seed in the center.

Hollow out a space in each avocado half, leaving most of the meat inside. This will be where your eggs sits, make sure there is enough room for the whole egg.

Crack one egg into each half of the avocado.

Sprinkle a little cheese on top of each avocado half.

Break up cooked bacon into small pieces, sprinkle over top of avocado.

Cook for about 15 minutes, or until warm and cheese is melted.

Egg and Sausage Casserole

Serves: 6-8 servings

Ingredients

1 pound ground breakfast sausage
2 cups shredded mozzarella cheese
6 large eggs
⅛ teaspoon salt
⅛ teaspoon pepper
⅛ teaspoon Italian seasoning or other desired spices

Instructions

Preheat oven to 350°F.
In an oiled skillet, brown the sausage. Drain excess fat.
Whisk eggs, seasonings and shredded cheese together in large mixing bowl.
Mix sausage and eggs and pour into a 9" pie pan.
Bake for about minutes or until firm.

Egg Breakfast Muffins

Ingredients
6 Eggs
1 green pepper (red/orange contain higher sugar content)
3 small onions or one large
1 large tomato
½ teaspoon salt

Instructions
Preheat the oven to 400°F.

Cut pepper, onions and tomatoes into small pieces, mix together in large mixing bowl.

Whisk eggs and seasonings together in another bowl, then pour over vegetable mixture.

Mix ingredients together so that vegetables are well dispersed in the eggs. Grease muffin tin (12 muffin) with cooking spray or olive oil to prevent egg from sticking.

Pour egg and vegetable mixture into muffin cups, making sure each tin has a uniform amount of egg and vegetable to avoid

uneven cooking.

Optional-add another sprinkle of cheese to the top, or add any other desired spices.

Bake for 15-18 minutes or until the tops are firm to the touch.

Let cool before serving. Store leftover cups in refrigerator or freezer.

Lunch Ideas

Keto Chicken Salad
2 cups chicken breast or dark meat, shredded
1/4 cup mayonnaise
1/2 cup sour cream
1 cup celery, chopped
1 cup sharp shredded cheddar cheese
1/4 cup yellow onion, minced
3 small green onions, sliced
1/2 c chopped bacon, from about 6 slices
Salt and pepper to taste

Instructions
Mix the chicken, celery, bacon, onions, and cheese in a large mixing bowl and mix in the mayonnaise and sour cream. Add salt and pepper to taste. Optional, add garlic powder, dried parsley or other spices to taste.

Mix well until everything is evenly coated and distributed throughout.

Chicken salad can be eaten plain or with low-carb bread or wraps or use to top a mixed green salad.

Low Carb Pizza

1½ cups shredded mozzarella cheese
¾ cup almond flour
2 tablespoons cream cheese
1 teaspoon white wine vinegar
1 egg
½ teaspoon salt
olive oil for coating pan

Topping

½ lb sweet or hot sausage
1 tablespoon butter
½ cup tomato sauce (must be unsweetened)
½ teaspoon dried oregano
1½ cups shredded mozzarella cheese
Preheat the oven to 400°F

Melt cream cheese and mozzarella cheese together. Stir until they melt together and uniform consistency. Add the other ingredients and mix well.

Oil your hands and flatten the dough on parchment paper or non stick pan, about 8 inches (20 cm) in diameter. A rolling pin may be helpful here, but is not necessary if it spreads evenly by hand.

Poke holes in the dough with a fork and bake for 10–12 minutes, or until golden brown.

While the dough is in the oven, brown the ground sausage meat in olive oil or butter. Optional-add minced onion for additional flavor.

Spread a thin layer of tomato sauce on crust. Add the meat and cheese.

Bake in middle of rack for 10-15 minutes or until crust and cheese are golden brown.

Serve with a mixed green salad.

**half pizza has 7 grams of carbs.

Low Carb Tuna Cheese Melt

2 pieces of low-carb bread (see recipe below)

Tuna Fish Salad
⅓ cup mayonnaise or sour cream
½ cup chopped celery
¼ cup chopped dill pickles
1 can tuna in olive oil or water
½ teaspoon lemon juice
½ minced garlic
salt and pepper, to taste

Topping
½ cup shredded cheddar cheese
1 pinch paprika

Low carb bread (makes 6-8)
3 eggs
½ cup cream cheese
1 pinch salt
½ tablespoon ground psyllium husk powder
½ teaspoon baking powder

Instructions

Preheat the oven to 350°F
Mix tuna salad ingredients together until uniform
Place the bread slices on a non-stick baking sheet. Spread the tuna mix on the bread and sprinkle cheese on top.
Add some paprika powder, or other desired spices.
Bake in oven until the cheese bubbles and turns golden brown. Top with leafy greens and drizzle with olive oil if desired.

Low Carb Bread **one slice of low carb bread has 2 grams of carbohydrate

Separate the eggs whites from yolks, keep yolks in a separate mixing bowl.
Whip egg whites together with salt until stiff peaks form. The whisked whites should be uniform consistency with no running.
Blend the egg yolks and cream cheese together. Add the psyllium seed husk and baking powder. Leave out for an airier, less bread-like consistency.
Mix the egg whites into the egg yolk mix – try to keep the air in the egg whites. Don't over stir.
Scoop mixture onto greased baking pan in 6-8 small clumps. These will bake into individual pieces.
Bake in the middle of the oven rack at 150° C for about 25 minutes or until the tops are light brown.

Avocado and Caprese Salad

Ingredients:
1/2 cup balsamic vinegar
1 tablespoon olive oil
2 tablespoons packed brown sugar
2 boneless chicken breasts, sliced thin
Salt and freshly ground black pepper, to taste
6 cups romaine lettuce, finely chopped
6 ounces fresh mozzarella
1 cup cherry tomatoes, cut in half
1 avocado, halved
1/4 cup basil leaves

Directions:
Add the balsamic vinegar and brown sugar to a small saucepan over medium heat. Bring to a slight boil and reduce by half. Let cool before serving.

Heat olive oil in a medium skillet over medium high heat.

Thinly slice chicken breast, making sure thickness is uniform. Season chicken breasts with salt and pepper, to taste. Place 2-3 pieces in the pan and cook, flipping once, until cooked through. Let cool before dicing into bite-size pieces.

Tear lettuce into a large bowl; top with chicken, cheese, tomatoes, avocado and spices. Drizzle the dressing on top of the salad and toss to combine.

Serve immediately, or store all ingredients in the refrigerator to serve cold. Great for making leftovers, sauté extra chicken for a second meal.

Lettuce Wraps with Turkey and Bacon

Ingredients

6 cups iceberg lettuce
4 slices turkey sliced
4 slices bacon, cooked
1 medium avocado, thinly sliced
1 roma tomato, thinly sliced

For the Spiced Mayo:
1/2 cup mayonnaise
6 large basil leaves, finely chopped, or 2 tbsp dried
1 tsp lemon juice
1 garlic clove, chopped
Salt and pepper to taste

Directions
For the Spiced Mayo: combine spices and mayonnaise in a food processor then blend until smooth.
Place two large lettuce leaves on a plate then add a slice of turkey to each leaf, and slather with Spiced Mayo. Layer on a second slice of turkey followed by the bacon, and a few slices of avocado and tomato. Add salt and pepper to taste, then fold like a taco. Slice in half then serve cold.

Dinner Ideas

Hamburger Patties with Creamy Tomato Sauce and Fried Cabbage

Hamburger patties

1½ lbs ground beef
1 egg
¼ cut feta cheese
1 teaspoon salt
¼ teaspoon ground black pepper
2 oz. fresh parsley, finely chopped
1 tablespoon olive oil
2 tbsps butter

Gravy

1¼ cups heavy whipping cream
2 tbsp fresh or dry parsley
2 tbsp tomato paste
Salt and pepper to taste

Fried green cabbage

1½ lbs shredded green cabbage
4 tbsp butter
Salt and pepper to taste

Instructions

Mix ground beef, cheese and spices for the hamburgers. When ingredients are uniform, form eight oblong patties.

Fry patties in a nonstick pan on medium high in both butter and olive oil until the patties are almost cooked to the desired level of doneness.

Pour the tomato paste and the whipping cream into the pan when the patties are almost done. Stir and let the cream boil together.

Butter-fried green cabbage

Shred the cabbage with a knife or food processor.

Melt butter in a frying pan.

Sauté the shredded cabbage on medium heat for at least 15 minutes or until the cabbage is wilted, and reaching the desired color and consistency.

Lower the heat a little towards the end. Stir regularly. Salt and pepper to taste.

Add parsley at the time of serving for garnish.

**11 grams of carbohydrates per serving

Chicken Breast with Herb Flavored Butter

Fried chicken
4 chicken breasts, butterflied or cut thin
2 tbsp. butter or olive oil
Salt and pepper to taste

Herb butter
½ cup butter, soft at room temperature
1 garlic clove
½ teaspoon garlic powder
¼ cup chopped fresh parsley
1 teaspoon lemon juice
½ teaspoon salt

Leafy greens
½ lb leafy greens, like dark romaine lettuce, spinach or kale

Instructions
Mix softened butter with spices for herb butter. Tip: Take butter out of the refrigerator about ½ hour before planning to prepare as to not need to soften using the microwave.

Mix together until spices are uniform in the butter. Set aside for later.

Season the chicken with salt and pepper. Fry in butter or oil on medium heat until the filets are cooked through.

Serve the chicken on a bed of leafy greens and add a generous amount of herb butter on top.

**1 gram of carbohydrate per serving

Broccoli and Cauliflower Gratin with Sweet Sausage

Serves 4

Ingredients

1 lb sweet sausage (or hot if desired)
1 leek
1 yellow onion
1 lb broccoli, chopped in large chunks.
½ lb cauliflower, chopped in large chunks.
2 tablespoons Dijon mustard
1 cup sour cream
4 oz. shredded cheese
2 tbsp butter
¼ cup fresh thyme
Salt and pepper, to taste

Instructions

Preheat the oven to 450°F
Chop vegetables and sausage.
Sautee onion and vegetables in butter in a nonstick pan. Add a little water to steam vegetables for quicker cooking.
 Brown the sweet sausage in a separate non-stick pan. May save some onion to sautee with sausage for added flavor.
Pour the vegetables in a baking dish, blend the mustard with the sour cream and pour over the vegetables. Make sure to cover all vegetables evenly.
Add the sausage and cheese on top and season with thyme.
Bake in oven on upper rack for 15 minutes or until top is golden brown.
***16 grams carbohydrate per serving**

Dessert Ideas

Low-Carb Molten Chocolate Cake

Ingredients

2 oz. dark chocolate with a minimum of 70% cocoa solids, as little added sugar as possible.

2 tbsp butter

¼ teaspoon vanilla extract

3 eggs

Instructions

Preheat your oven to 400°F. and grease

Coat 4-6 small ramekins with butter or oil

Break the chocolate into small pieces. Melt with the butter carefully on medium heat. Watch carefully, as chocolate burns easily.

Stir into a smooth batter and add the vanilla. Turn off the heat and set aside. Let the chocolate cool, but should not solidify.

Whisk eggs in a bowl with a hand mixer for 2-3 minutes until fluffy.

Pour in the chocolate batter. Mix well, preferably with a wooden spoon or fork, until the batter is smooth.

Pour the batter into the greased ramekins and bake in the oven. As soon as they are in, lower the heat to 350°F.

Bake for 5–7 minutes, depending on number of servings.

Remove from the oven and serve warm. May add cream cheese on top for added flavor.

Coconut and Chocolate Bars

Ingredients

1 cup shredded coconut (must be unsweetened)
1 packet of no calorie sweetener
1 tsp vanilla extract
⅓ cup coconut cream (unsweetened)
4 tbsp coconut oil
2 tbsp unsweetened cocoa powder

Instructions

Mix the coconut, coconut cream,1/2 of the vanilla extract and ½ packet of sweetener and blend well in a mixing bowl.

Place all of the shredded coconut mixture on a small non-stick cookie sheet.

Shape the mixture into a one-inch thick square, making sure thickness is uniform throughout.

Place in the freezer until frozen solid. Best to do this overnight.

Mix coconut oil in a small sauce pan until liquefied

Add cocoa powder, ½ packet of sweetener and vanilla extract to the melted coconut oil

Mix well on low heat for about 2 minutes, until all ingredients are well blended

Let cool to room temperature, but still liquid

Remove from the freezer and cut into 5 bars

Drop the bars in the cocoa liquid, and submerge all sides to coat evenly.

Place bars back on the cookie sheet or tray

When all bars are all coated put in the refrigerator to harden.

Store the bars in the fridge for harder product or at room temperature for softer, just remember that the chocolate will melt if room temperature is too high.

Conclusion

Thanks for making it through to the end of this book, let's hope it was informative and able to provide you with all of the tools you need to become a fat burning machine!

The next step is to start the Ketogenic Diet. Use this guide to get organized and prepared for success!

Finally, if you found this book useful in anyway, a review on Amazon is always appreciated!